INTRODUCTION

A Special Statutory Funding Program for Type 1 Diabetes Research is mandated by Section 330B of the Public Health Service Act. This program was initially established by Section 4921 of the Balanced Budget Act of 1997 (P.L. 105-33) and later extended and augmented by Section 931 of the 2001 Consolidated Appropriations Act (P.L. 106-554) and by the Public Health Service Act Amendment for Diabetes (P.L. 107-360). Section 330B states:

Sec. 330B. [254c-2] Special Diabetes Programs for Type 1 Diabetes

"(a) In General. – The Secretary, directly or through grants, shall provide for research into the prevention and cure of Type 1 diabetes."

"(b) Funding.–

(1) Transferred Funds. – Notwithstanding section 2140(a) of the Social Security Act, from the amounts appropriated in such section for each of the fiscal years 1998 through 2002, $30,000,000 is hereby transferred and made available in such fiscal years for grants under this section."

"(2) Appropriations. – For the purpose of making grants under this section, there is appropriated, out of any funds in the Treasury not otherwise appropriated –

(A) $70,000,000 for each of fiscal years 2001 and 2002 (which shall be combined with amounts transferred under paragraph (1) for each such fiscal years);

(B) $100,000,000 for fiscal year 2003; and

(C) $150,000,000 for fiscal years 2004 through 2008."

This program also has mandated reporting requirements to the Congress. Section 4923 of the Balanced Budget Act of 1997, as amended by section 931 of the FY 2001 Consolidated Appropriations Act and by Section 1(c) of the Public Health Service Act Amendment for Diabetes, states:

Report on Diabetes Grant Programs

"(a) Evaluation. – The Secretary of Health and Human Services shall conduct an evaluation of the diabetes grant programs established under the amendments made by this chapter."

"(b) Reports. – The Secretary shall submit to the appropriate committees of Congress –

(1) an interim report on the evaluation conducted under subsection (a) not later than January 1, 2000, and

(2) a final report on such evaluation not later than January 1, 2007."

The first mandated interim report was transmitted to the Congress in 2000. The current report, which has been prepared by the National Institute of Diabetes and Digestive and Kidney Diseases (NIDDK), National Institutes of Health (NIH), Department of Health and Human Services (DHHS), was initially prepared to meet a January 2003 statutory reporting requirement to the Congress on this program. That reporting requirement has now been changed to January 2007, as a result of the President's signature into law of P.L. 107-360. The NIDDK is proceeding to issue the current report because it provides an important interim assessment of the program by external scientific experts, grant recipients, and NIDDK staff who have analyzed the associated scientific literature and other relevant data on the program. Moreover, the report contains a highly useful summary of research opportunities identified by external experts in the field. These opportunities can thus serve as a scientific guidepost in developing this program in the years ahead.

REPORT ON PROGRESS
& OPPORTUNITIES:
EXECUTIVE SUMMARY

Special Statutory
Funding Program for
Type 1 Diabetes
Research

This booklet summarizes a document entitled "Special
Statutory Funding Program for Type 1 Diabetes Research:
Report on Progress & Opportunities." The entire document
can be found at http://www.niddk.nih.gov/ under the
"Reports, Testimony, and Plans" section.

April 2003

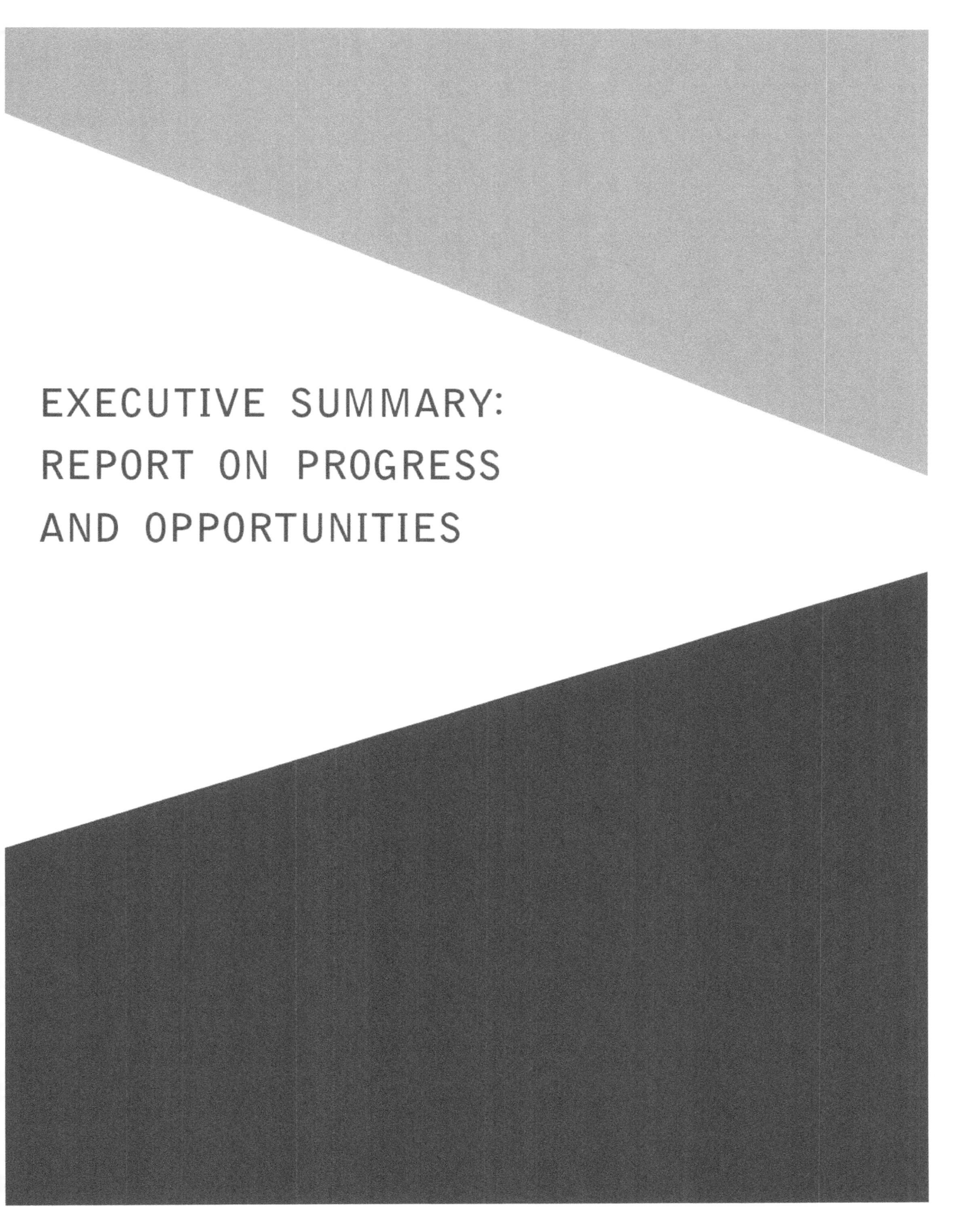

EXECUTIVE SUMMARY: REPORT ON PROGRESS AND OPPORTUNITIES

Type 1 diabetes—also known as juvenile diabetes—is a devastating illness that often strikes in childhood or adolescence. The afflicted individual's own immune system mistakenly attacks and destroys the beta cells of the pancreatic islets, which are the sole producers of insulin. If left untreated, this disease results in death from starvation despite high levels of glucose (sugar) in the bloodstream; without insulin, the tissues of the body cannot absorb or use glucose, the major cellular fuel. The discovery and purification of insulin by a team of medical researchers at the University of Toronto in 1921 quickly led to the realization that this pancreatic hormone was the key to restoring the body's ability to process glucose. This insight, which was recognized by the award of a Nobel Prize, provided a life-saving treatment for type 1 diabetes in the form of daily insulin injections.

Insulin therapy—while life-supporting—is not a cure for those with type 1 diabetes, who represent an estimated 5 to 10 percent of the 11.1 million Americans with diagnosed diabetes[1]. Moreover, the treatment regimen for this disease requires constant attention and is difficult to maintain even in the best of circumstances. On a daily basis, individuals with type 1 diabetes must balance multiple insulin injections or an insulin pump—and frequent finger sticks to test blood sugar levels—in conjunction with their food intake and physical exercise. Even the most vigilant patients are at risk for sudden, acute episodes of dangerously low or high blood glucose levels (*hypo*glycemia or *hyper*glycemia, respectively), either of which can be life-threatening in extreme cases.

Persistent elevation of blood glucose levels, despite insulin therapy, slowly damages nearly all of the body's organs, including the eyes, kidneys and urologic tract, nerves, and cardiovascular system. Type 1 diabetes substantially increases the risk of blindness, kidney failure, chronic wounds and skin ulcers, nerve pain and other neurological problems, limb amputation, heart disease and heart attacks, stroke, high blood pressure, gum disease, and pregnancy-related problems. Due to these serious, long-term complications, type 1 diabetes reduces quality-of-life and is estimated to shorten the average life span by 15 years. Individuals with another, more common form of diabetes—type 2 diabetes—face a similar risk of severe complications, although the disease processes underlying type 1 and type 2 diabetes are different.

1 Another 5.9 million Americans are estimated to have undiagnosed diabetes—bringing the total number of diabetes patients in the U.S. to 17 million.

By 1998, when the Special Statutory Funding Program for Type 1 Diabetes Research was launched, important advances in medical research had opened up exciting new leads in the search for methods to prevent and cure this disease and its complications. The success of the Human Genome Project greatly accelerated the pace of genetics research to identify new disease-related genes. A burgeoning knowledge of the immune system made it feasible to devise innovative strategies to prevent or reverse the autoimmune process at the heart of type 1 diabetes. Such research now underpins clinical trials of promising immunoprevention strategies for blocking the onset or progression of disease, and progress in islet transplantation research. Advances in molecular and cellular biology fostered an integrated approach to understanding the development and biology of the insulin-producing pancreatic beta cell, which is central to diabetes pathology. The Diabetes Control and Complications Trial, which ended in 1993, demonstrated that tight control of blood glucose through intensive insulin therapy could significantly reduce or delay many diabetic complications. This landmark finding spurred a paradigm shift in the daily management of type 1 diabetes and has energized research on new approaches to improve therapy of type 1 diabetes. Perhaps most importantly, a recent study[2] of type 1 diabetic individuals in Allegheny County, Pennsylvania, revealed that death rates between 10 and 20 years after diagnosis had fallen from 8.4 percent in patients diagnosed in the 1965-1969 period to 3.5 percent in those diagnosed in the period of 1975-1979. Thus, research advances in the medical care of diabetes —such as self-monitoring of blood glucose and better management of blood pressure—are making a measurable, positive difference in patients' lives.

In short, the Special Statutory Funding Program for Type 1 Diabetes Research began at an opportune time for the scientific community to capitalize on new research technologies and findings and apply them to type 1 diabetes. The special statutory funding program has continued, throughout the first 5 years, to promote focused, innovative, and clinically-relevant research that has enabled significant progress to be made toward understanding, preventing, and, ultimately, curing type 1 diabetes and its complications. Particularly after the increase in special statutory funding in FY 2001, large-scale, collaborative research programs have been established that could not otherwise have been under-taken—or at least not at a scientifically optimal scale. Importantly, the diabetes research and voluntary communities—which have been essential partners at every stage of the special statutory funding program— have been energized by the scientific advances supported by the program, and have identified critical new oppor-tunities now emerging from this targeted investment in type 1 diabetes research.

2 Nishimura, R., R.E. LaPorte, J.S. Dorman, N. Tajima, D. Becker, and T.J. Orchard. 2001. Mortality trends in type 1 diabetes. Diabetes Care 24:823-828.

OVERVIEW OF THE SPECIAL STATUTORY FUNDING PROGRAM FOR TYPE 1 DIABETES RESEARCH

Special funding for type 1 diabetes research, in the total amount of $1.14 billion for FY 1998 through FY 2008, was provided to the Secretary of Health and Human Services through Section 330B of the Public Health Service Act. The original enabling legislation was the Balanced Budget Act of 1997 (Public Law 105-33), which was later amended by the FY 2001 Consolidated Appropriations Act (Public Law 106-554) and by the Public Health Service Act Amendment for Diabetes (Public Law 107-360) to extend the special statutory funding program in time and amount (Table 1). This funding program augments regularly appropriated funds that the Department of Health and Human Services (HHS) receives for diabetes research through the Labor-HHS-Education Appropriations Committees. The National Institute of Diabetes and Digestive and Kidney Diseases (NIDDK), through authority granted by the Secretary, has a leadership role in planning, implementing, and evaluating the allocation of these funds.

TABLE 1 **Special Statutory Funds for Type 1 Diabetes Research–in Millions of Dollars**

FY	1998	1999	2000	2001	2002	2003	2004	2005	2006	2007	2008	Total
P.L. 105-33	30	30	30	30	30	—	—	—	—	—	—	150
P.L. 106-554	—	—	—	70	70	100	—	—	—	—	—	240
P.L. 107-360	—	—	—	—	—	—	150	150	150	150	150	750
TOTAL	**30**	**30**	**30**	**100**	**100**	**100**	**150**	**150**	**150**	**150**	**150**	**1,140**

From its inception in FY 1998, the Special
Statutory Funding Program for Type 1 Diabetes
Research has achieved:

- An innovative paradigm for trans-HHS, cross-disciplinary research planning and management that benefits from the wide range of scientific expertise on type 1 diabetes within the NIH, CDC, and other HHS components;

- Active involvement of the external diabetes research and voluntary communities throughout the planning, implementation, and evaluation phases of the program;

- A scientifically-focused, but flexible, budgeting process that allows a rapid response to emerging research topics of critical importance;

- Establishment of large-scale, collaborative, and infrastructural initiatives that extend beyond the scope of traditional research programs and maximize investment by focusing the talent, insights, and resources of many scientists on common research questions;

- Promotion of diverse, innovative, and high-impact research, which emphasizes both clinical research with the potential to improve the lives of diabetes patients and basic research that will provide the fundamental knowledge necessary to develop the next generation of treatment strategies;

- Emphasis on recruitment and support of new investigators and "new-to-diabetes" researchers with varied expertise and access to state-of-the-art technologies;

- Advancement of research that will accelerate the understanding, prevention, treatment, and cure of type 1 diabetes through innovative technologies, new targets for drug development, and novel therapeutic strategies to combat the disease and its complications.

Planning Process

To ensure the most scientifically productive use of the special statutory funds, the NIDDK initiated a collaborative planning process that involves the participation of the relevant institutes and centers of the NIH, including the National Center for Research Resources (NCRR), National Eye Institute (NEI), National Human Genome Research Institute (NHGRI), National Heart, Lung, and Blood Institute (NHLBI), National Institute of Allergy and Infectious Diseases (NIAID), National Institute of Child Health and Human Development (NICHD), National Institute of Dental and Craniofacial Research (NIDCR), National Institute of Environmental Health Sciences (NIEHS), National Institute of Neurological Disorders and Stroke (NINDS), National Institute of Nursing Research (NINR), National Library of Medicine (NLM), and other NIH institutes and centers that are represented on the Diabetes Mellitus Interagency Coordinating Committee, the Centers for Disease Control and Prevention (CDC), the Agency for Health Care Research and Quality (AHRQ), the Food and Drug Administration (FDA), and the two major diabetes voluntary organizations: the Juvenile Diabetes Research Foundation International (JDRF) and the American Diabetes Association (ADA).

Critical to the planning process is scientific advice the NIH has garnered from the type 1 diabetes research community. Sources of input include a variety of scientific workshops and conferences; the recommendations in the 5-year plan of the independent, congressionally-established Diabetes Research Working Group; the advice of a group of distinguished scientists who convened in April 2000 to consider opportunities for allocation of the special statutory funds; and the recommendations of a panel of scientific experts who met in May 2002 to evaluate the use of the special statutory funds and assess opportunities for future research.

Implementation of the Special Statutory Funding Program

The special statutory funds have been expended through a variety of mechanisms in response to recommendations of the trans-HHS planning groups and external advisory panels. Large-scale consortia have been launched to support multidisciplinary, collaborative research projects that benefit from the input of scientists with wide-ranging expertise. These consortia, as well as newly-established research resources, expand the scope and power of research efforts by making technological developments and tools available to broad segments of the type 1 diabetes research community. Thus, they foster research that would be difficult to achieve in a timely fashion in individual laboratories. The special funding program has also solicited investigator-initiated research on topics of urgent and unmet need, such as diabetic nerve disease (neuropathy) and other issues of importance to the prevention and cure of type 1 diabetes and its complications, through announcements known as "Requests for Applications" or "RFAs." The special program has emphasized the use of R21 pilot and feasibility awards. The R21 mechanism supports short-term grants for innovative, high-risk/high-impact research. A limited number of administrative supplements were also made to existing research grants or programs to facilitate rapid action in response to emerging scientific opportunities of critical importance. By not building up a commitment base for multi-year funding, these 1-year supplements have helped to maintain budgeting flexibility in the later years of the special funding program.

Evaluation Process

The public laws providing the special statutory funds also mandate interim and final evaluation reports on the use of the funds. Initiatives pursued with the Public Law 105-33 funds are described in a 2000 report to the Congress, which is available on the NIDDK website (http://www.niddk.nih.gov/federal/initiative.htm). This interim evaluation report describes the collaborative, trans-HHS planning process that guides the use of the special funds, the objectives and expected accomplishments of research programs and resources that have been established, and scientific advances achieved through the early initiatives. Research progress and opportunities that have resulted from the special funding program from FY 1998 through 2003 are highlighted. A final mandated evaluation report will be sent to the Congress in January 2007.

Critical assessment of the planning and implementation process, and of the scientific merit of the Special Statutory Funding Program for Type 1 Diabetes Research, has been garnered through an evaluation process involving the external diabetes research community, as well as an internal review of archival data. Especially important to this process has been a professional assessment of the special statutory funding program, which was rendered by an advisory panel of scientific experts on type 1 diabetes, convened at the NIH in May 2002. This panel reviewed the use of the special statutory funds and identified opportunities for future scientific research that have emerged from recent progress in the type 1 diabetes field. Moreover, a survey was conducted of extramural researchers, who received grants awarded with the special statutory funds from FY 1998 through 2000, to gather information about scientific advances that resulted from the special funding, and about the impact of this program on grantees' research and careers. The findings of this Office of Management and Budget (OMB)-approved survey reflect the self-reported, professional judgments and opinions of the program's grantees. Finally, archival sources within the NIH and CDC were examined to assess the allocation of the special statutory funds, the outcomes of research solicitations, the recruitment of researchers to the diabetes field, and publications and other measures of scientific advances attributable to the special statutory funding program.

These various assessment measures indicate that the Special Statutory Funding Program for Type 1 Diabetes Research has been highly effective and productive to date. However, it is not yet possible to assess the long-term impact that this special program will have on the diabetes research field, given that many new initiatives were first launched in FY 2001 and 2002, funds for FY 2003 have yet to be fully deployed, and planning for FY 2004 through 2008 is just beginning.

PURSUIT OF SIX MAJOR SCIENTIFIC GOALS: PROGRAM EFFORTS AND ACHIEVEMENTS

The Special Statutory Funding Program for Type 1 Diabetes Research has been framed around the following six broad, scientific goals:

Goal I: Identify the Genetic and Environmental Causes of Type 1 Diabetes

A complex interplay of genetic and environmental factors underlies the development of type 1 diabetes. Variations in a large DNA region containing immune system genes—the major histocompatibility HLA[3] class II locus—account for about half of the genetic susceptibility to type 1 diabetes. As many as 20 other stretches of DNA are suspected, but thus far not proven, to contain genes that influence the development of type 1 diabetes. Likewise, environmental factors— such as viral infections, diet, or other factors to which fetuses, infants, and children are exposed—that may trigger disease in genetically susceptible individuals, have remained elusive. Identifying the causes of disease susceptibility is essential for understanding the molecular mechanisms of type 1 diabetes, developing new targets for drug development, and improving early identification and prevention strategies in at-risk individuals. Accomplishing this goal requires the cooperative efforts of many investigators. The Special Statutory Funding Program for Type 1 Diabetes Research has allowed the establishment of resource-sharing consortia whose members can pool expertise, data, technologies, and, perhaps most important, access to large patient populations beyond the scope of individual laboratories.

3 Human Leukocyte Antigens (HLA) are genetically-determined molecules on the surface of all cells in the body. The HLA system assures that the immune system recognizes the individual's own tissues as self rather than foreign. In people susceptible to type 1 diabetes, this recognition system goes awry and produces an autoimmune response to insulin-producing beta cells.

Although clinical symptoms of type 1 diabetes can appear abruptly, research has shown that the decline of beta cell function occurs over a long period of time prior to disease onset. For this reason, the ability to identify at-risk individuals is critical. The recently completed first phase of the Diabetes Prevention Trial for Type 1 Diabetes (DPT-1) (*see also Goal II*), which screened approximately 100,000 relatives of type 1 diabetes patients, showed that researchers could accurately predict which of those relatives had a 50 percent risk of developing type 1 diabetes within 5 years. The researchers used a combination of genetic, metabolic, and immunologic markers to make those determinations. This landmark result will be an invaluable aid in the design of future trials of novel prevention strategies.

The ongoing search for additional genetic predictors of type 1 diabetes has been newly energized by the launch of the International Type 1 Diabetes Genetics Consortium. This team of investigators from the U.S., Europe, and Australia has the capacity to collect the large number of patient samples necessary to perform genome-wide screens for diabetes susceptibility genes. A related effort, the International Histocompatibility Working Group, is looking for single DNA subunit changes in candidate susceptibility genes. The frequency of such changes in the population may help researchers define gene variants that contribute to diabetes risk. A genetics component of the Epidemiology of Diabetic Interventions and Complications (EDIC) Study has begun to search for genes conferring susceptibility to diabetic complications, such as eye and kidney disease. Although the EDIC patient group is relatively small— approximately 1,400 type 1 diabetic patients and their close relatives—these dedicated study volunteers have been extensively characterized for nearly 20 years, since their participation in the Diabetes Control and

Complications Trial (DCCT). The EDIC genetics study is expected to provide crucial insights regarding the underlying mechanisms of diabetic complications.

By bringing together a multidisciplinary, international group of investigators, the Triggers and Environmental Determinants of Diabetes in Youth (TEDDY) consortium provides a coordinated approach to the search for non-genetic factors contributing to type 1 diabetes. The scale of this consortium ensures optimal analysis of gene-environment interactions and the inclusion of individuals from diverse ethnic backgrounds. These efforts are complemented by an epidemiological study associated with the Type 1 Diabetes TrialNet—a nation-wide network of clinical trial centers for type 1 diabetes (*see also Goal II*). The large number of relatives of type 1 diabetes patients who will be screened through TrialNet represents a unique opportunity to follow the natural history and progression of disease and to potentially uncover environmental triggers. The SEARCH program, a joint effort of the CDC and NIH, is identifying all forms of diabetes in children within defined U.S. populations. The results of SEARCH will help to standardize the ascertainment of childhood diabetes and document the burden of this disease in young patients.

Research to locate and study genes and other factors that cause type 1 diabetes in humans benefits from expanded basic studies in animal models. A mouse repository has been established to ensure survival of type 1 diabetes model strains and to facilitate distribution of these valuable research tools to investigators. Efforts to sequence susceptibility genes in one such strain—the non-obese diabetic (NOD) mouse model of type 1 diabetes—will accelerate the search for parallel genes in humans.

While much work remains to be done, initiatives launched through the special statutory funding program have positioned the diabetes genetics and epidemiology research communities to carry out well-coordinated studies with sufficient statistical power for identifying genetic and environmental triggers of type 1 diabetes and its complications. The results of these investigations on the underlying causes of disease will inform and advance other fields of research on new methods to prevent, treat, and cure type 1 diabetes.

Goal II: Prevent or Reverse Type 1 Diabetes

Immune-mediated destruction of the insulin-producing pancreatic beta cells results in type 1 diabetes. Defining the molecular defects that provoke the immune system to mistakenly attack and destroy the beta cells is key to the development of methods to prevent or reverse this "autoimmune" process. In particular, strategies to establish immune tolerance[4] have the potential to block autoimmunity in at-risk individuals and to facilitate transplantation of new pancreatic islets from organ donors that could potentially cure this disease in those already afflicted. The Special Statutory Funding Program for Type 1 Diabetes Research supports a broad spectrum of research on autoimmunity and its treatment, including clinical studies in at-risk or new-onset patients, preclinical work on the fundamental mechanisms of the immune system, and the development of resources that facilitate the work of the entire diabetes research community.

---

4 Immune tolerance is the process by which the immune system accepts a foreign substance—such as a transplanted islet or an injected protein—as "self" and no longer mounts a destructive response against it.

Central to type 1 diabetes research is the design of a "vaccine" or drug that can prevent disease in susceptible individuals or reverse autoimmunity in new-onset patients who still retain residual beta cell function. The DPT-1 (*see also Goal I*) tested—and disproved— the theory that the injection of low doses of insulin could block the onset of the disease in genetically-at-risk persons. Although this was not the hoped-for result, the findings of this major clinical trial will spare many from an ineffective, burdensome "therapy" that was already in use by some physicians. A second trial of the DPT-1 is testing the efficacy of oral application of insulin, which interacts with the immune system through a mechanism different from that of injected insulin. This research is in progress through the Type 1 Diabetes TrialNet (*see also Goal I*). An international network of clinical centers, investigators, and core laboratory facilities, TrialNet is poised to evaluate new therapeutic agents for type 1 diabetes prevention in human patients. The international scale of TrialNet and the availability of extensive scientific expertise and core resources are designed to expedite pilot testing of promising new treatment strategies that, if successful, can quickly be moved to larger clinical trials. A complementary initiative, the Immune Tolerance Network (ITN) (*see also Goal III*), studies immunosuppressive agents that selectively block the autoimmune process of type 1 diabetes, or impede immune-mediated rejection of transplanted islets without repressing the entire immune system. In a small preliminary study, treatment with a monoclonal antibody targeted at T cells implicated in autoimmunity was able to preserve insulin production in newly diagnosed type 1 diabetes patients for at least 12 months after diagnosis. The ITN, an international collaboration of basic and clinical scientists, will expand testing of this promising therapy to a larger patient population with new onset type 1 diabetes. If successful, TrialNet will expand the study of this treatment for use in preventing disease in at-risk individuals. Another clinical study, the Trial to Reduce the Incidence of Type 1 Diabetes in the Genetically-At-Risk (TRIGR), is investigating a specific hypothesis of disease prevention—that breaking down the proteins in cow's milk formula can reduce the incidence of antibodies directed against beta cell antigens associated with the subsequent development of type 1 diabetes in infants who are at high risk of this disease because of their genetic background.

The rational design of novel therapeutic agents and strategies depends on preclinical research to elucidate the molecular mechanisms of the immune system and identify new targets for intervention. Scientists have developed new animal models that carry human immune system genes or have alterations in other proteins suspected of involvement in type 1 diabetes pathogenesis. These important research tools help to advance our understanding of how the immune system works normally and how it goes awry in type 1 diabetes. Autoimmune Disease Prevention Centers have been established to promote basic and preclinical research on the mechanisms that underlie autoimmune diseases, including type 1 diabetes. This collaborative group of investigators focuses on prevention of autoimmunity by methods other than global immunosuppression, which leaves the patient vulnerable to infectious diseases and other medical problems.

Several initiatives have been launched to aid the conduct of type 1 diabetes prevention research. A program to standardize the measurement of diabetes autoantibodies, which is crucial to the prediction of disease risk, has helped to minimize laboratory variability in these assays. Likewise, an effort is under way to standardize the C-peptide[5] assay that clinical trial researchers use to assess the efficacy of autoimmune prevention strategies. A central repository for data and biologic samples collected during clinical trials provides an opportunity for scientists to maximize the value of these trials by proposing ancillary research studies that were not included in original trial designs. Multiple consortia, including TrialNet and the ITN, as well as research networks aligned with other type 1 diabetes research goals, will benefit from this repository.

---

5 C-peptide refers to a small protein fragment that is released into the bloodstream when insulin is processed in the beta cells. Because insulin that diabetic individuals inject to control their blood glucose levels does not contain C-peptide, this fragment can serve as a marker of how much insulin is being produced by the pancreas and, thus, how well the beta cells are functioning.

Clinical researchers are moving quickly to develop and test novel, highly-specific strategies for the induction of immune tolerance and prevention of autoimmunity. The major trial networks that are supported by the special statutory funding program are invaluable for moving fundamental scientific discoveries to the bedside of patients who can potentially benefit. Moreover, preclinical and basic research on the immune system, which is a key component of the special funding program, provides the foundation for the design of new treatment regimens for the prevention of type 1 diabetes.

Goal III: Develop Cell Replacement Therapy

Pancreatic beta cells continuously sense the amount of glucose in the blood and release enough insulin to maintain that glucose level within a narrowly defined, optimal range. Strategies to replace beta cells that have been lost to autoimmune destruction would free type 1 diabetes patients from the need for external glucose monitoring and insulin delivery. Moreover, replacement cells would achieve tighter glucose control than is currently possible with insulin therapy and, thus, reduce the development of diabetic complications. The Special Statutory Funding Program for Type 1 Diabetes Research is vigorously pursuing a variety of research activities to understand the basic biology of the beta cells and to optimize new therapeutic approaches to beta cell replacement.

Understanding the development of beta cells and the molecular details of their specialized functions could lead, in the long term, to the development of renewable sources of beta cells that can be grown in a laboratory in unlimited quantities and transplanted into patients to potentially cure type 1 diabetes. Scientists have identified proteins that determine, in the early stages of pancreas development, whether progenitor cells proceed down a pathway of beta cell differentiation or become another pancreatic cell type. Investigators are also making progress in isolating multipotent stem cells that can differentiate into a variety of cells; research is under way to define conditions that selectively direct such stem cells towards beta cell differentiation. An international group of researchers, the Beta Cell Biology

Consortium, is working together to explore beta cell development and to apply the knowledge they gain to the generation of renewable beta cells. In a related effort, teams of investigators are studying molecular signaling pathways within individual beta cells, and between the beta cells and other components of the pancreas. The research undertaken through these programs will benefit from the development of a microarray chip that was designed to contain genes expressed in the pancreas or implicated in diabetes. This valuable research tool, which is available to the entire diabetes research community, enables researchers to simultaneously track changes in the expression of thousands of beta cell genes during varying developmental stages or physiological conditions.

While the generation of renewable sources of beta cells holds immense promise for the future, great strides are currently being made in the transplantation of donor islets, which are small clusters within the pancreas comprised of beta cells and other hormone-secreting cells. A recent breakthrough in this field occurred through research performed at the University of Alberta in Edmonton, Canada. The so-called "Edmonton protocol" of islet transplantation has led to long-term insulin independence for many type 1 diabetes patients who received infusions of donor islets. These patients, although free of the need for insulin therapy, must take immunosuppressive drugs for the rest of their lives to prevent immune rejection of the new islets. The special statutory funding program is actively pursuing a continuum of research and resource development efforts to refine and expand islet transplantation procedures. A Non-Human Primate Immune Tolerance Cooperative Study Group is performing preclinical development and testing of new protocols for immune suppression in transplant recipients. Ideally, the next generation of immunomodulatory agents will be able to selectively protect islet or other organ grafts from immune attack without subjecting the patient to the harsh side effects associated with current suppression therapy. The Collaborative Islet Transplant Registry has been established to collect information on all clinical trials with human patients in the U.S. or Canada to improve methods of islet engraftment, survival, and function. This registry will enable the transplantation research community to work synergistically on advancing the efficacy and availability of this promising therapy. Clinical investigation on human islets is being facilitated by new Islet Cell Resource Centers that provide human islets isolated under strict sterility conditions for transplantation research. By developing new harvesting techniques to improve the quality of isolated islets, these facilities will also contribute to efforts to maximize the number of patients who can receive transplants.

The recent progress in islet transplantation holds out real hope for a cure for type 1 diabetes, but several obstacles must be overcome before this treatment is suitable and available for all type 1 diabetic individuals. The special statutory funding program reflects a strong commitment to meeting the remaining challenges by increasing knowledge about beta cell biology, applying these new insights to the development of a renewable source of beta cells, and optimizing the islet isolation, surgical, and immunosuppression technologies that are needed to bring the promise of a cure to all type 1 diabetes patients.

Goal IV: Prevent or Reduce Hypoglycemia in Type 1 Diabetes

Individuals with type 1 diabetes must vigilantly guard against episodes of hypoglycemia—dangerously low blood glucose—that can result in symptoms ranging from dizziness to coma or death. Hypoglycemia can occur suddenly, brought on by an imbalance in insulin injections, food intake, and physical activity. An excess of insulin circulating in the blood causes glucose levels to drop precipitously below the level that is necessary to sustain the body's functions. Even highly motivated patients, who diligently manage their diabetes, are at risk of an acute hypoglycemic episode that can be caused by intensive insulin therapy. In some cases, patients may lose the ability to sense falling glucose levels— a condition known as "hypoglycemia unawareness"— which puts them at heightened risk of serious outcomes. Little is known at a molecular or cellular level about the

causes of hypoglycemia unawareness. The neuroscience underlying this condition has been a difficult area of research. The Special Statutory Funding Program for Type 1 Diabetes Research promotes research on new approaches to mitigate hypoglycemia and supports the development of new technologies for improved glucose monitoring and insulin delivery.

The Diabetes Control and Complications Trial (DCCT) demonstrated that intensive insulin therapy to closely control blood glucose levels reduces the risk of long-term diabetic complications such as blindness and kidney failure in type 1 diabetes patients, but increases the number of acute hypoglycemic events, at least in adults and children older than 13 years of age. The potential risks to younger children of increased hypoglycemia have impeded the implementation of intensive insulin therapy in this population. A clinical research consortium, DirecNet, has been established to test continuous glucose sensing technology in young children to determine whether new devices can help reduce the risk of hypoglycemia and improve glucose control in children. DirecNet investigators will also study glucose values in both children with type 1 diabetes and non-diabetic children to determine the normal range of blood glucose levels and the frequency of hypoglycemia in these groups. This research is expected to provide new insights for optimizing the management of diabetes in very young children.

Currently, diabetes management required patients to perform multiple, painful finger sticks each day to carefully monitor blood glucose levels. Glucose levels in the interstitial fluid between skin cells are now being studied as a surrogate for blood glucose measurements. Accessing the interstitial fluid has the potential to provide a more frequent and less painful method of glucose measurement than a finger stick to draw blood. In addition, researchers are exploring novel approaches that use minimally- or non-invasive technology to measure glucose. New continuous glucose sensing devices may incorporate signals to warn a patient of impending hypoglycemia, or link to an insulin delivery system to provide seamless metabolic control. These efforts are complemented by research to explore the brain's mechanisms for sensing glucose levels and mounting a counter-regulatory response.

Hypoglycemia is an extremely distressing condition for type 1 diabetic patients and is especially problematic in young children, who may not be able to recognize or communicate that an episode is occurring. The special statutory funding program is committed to supporting research to address the underlying causes and effective treatments of hypoglycemia. New initiatives in the neuroscience of hypoglycemia and hypoglycemia unawareness are laying the foundation for future clinical research. Moreover, research on cutting-edge technologies for sensing glucose and regulating insulin delivery, complemented by clinical trials to apply these advances to diabetes management in children, will help to improve the quality-of-life of type 1 diabetes patients.

Goal V: Prevent or Reduce the Complications of Type 1 Diabetes

Despite vigilant glucose monitoring and insulin therapy, type 1 diabetes patients often exhibit hyperglycemia—blood glucose levels that are significantly higher than normal. Chronic hyperglycemia slowly damages nearly every organ in the body. Over time, this condition can lead to serious complications, including blindness, kidney failure, and severe nerve pain, among other problems. Diabetic complications—which are common to both type 1 and type 2 diabetes—constitute a significant public health burden due to the reduction of patient health and quality-of-life, as well as the considerable costs to the health care system from treating these conditions. The Special Statutory Funding Program for Type 1 Diabetes Research is undertaking several major initiatives to find new strategies for combating the long-term health consequences of type 1 diabetes.

Some individuals are genetically predisposed to developing certain diabetic complications, such as retinopathy (eye disease) or nephropathy (kidney disease). Genetic factors involved in these complications have not been identified, nor is it yet known whether the same genes contribute to susceptibility to both eye and kidney disease or if distinct gene variants are uniquely involved in different complications. The Genetics of Kidneys in Diabetes (GoKinD) Study has been launched to examine the effects of genetics on the development of diabetic kidney disease in type 1 diabetes patients. This study will facilitate the collection of samples from the large number of patients required to track the genetic components of kidney disease. A related effort, the Family Investigation of Nephropathy and Diabetes (FIND) Study, is looking for genetic associations of diabetic kidney disease in both type 1 and type 2 diabetes patients. The special statutory funds enabled the addition of a second component to this study for the investigation of the genetic causes of diabetic eye disease. Both GoKinD and FIND are expected to reveal new targets for the development of therapies to prevent or treat the devastating complications of diabetes.

Clinical research and trials on new methods to reduce the incidence of or treat diabetic complications are under way on several fronts. Tight glucose control through intensive insulin therapy has already been demonstrated to decrease eye, nerve, and kidney-related complications of diabetes. The impact of this regimen on cardiovascular disease and stroke and on urologic health is now being assessed in the well-characterized EDIC study cohort (*see also Goal I*). A newly-established research consortium, the Diabetic Macular Edema Clinical Trials Network, is evaluating novel strategies for the treatment of diabetic eye disease. In addition, pilot trials are being undertaken to investigate potential therapies designed to slow or block the progression of diabetic kidney disease.

The groundwork for future clinical studies is being laid by basic research to uncover the molecular mechanisms through which high glucose affects tissue function. A collaborative research group, the Animal Models of Diabetic Complications Consortium (AMDCC), has been formed to derive and validate animal models that mimic human diabetic complications. Such models will be invaluable for understanding the biology of diabetic complications, as well as for the development and testing of potential new screening or diagnostic methods, prevention strategies, and pharmaceutical agents to reduce the burden of disease. Researchers are also searching for surrogate markers or imaging technologies that can detect the early stages of complications. Such markers would provide endpoints that could allow clinical trials to be conducted in a more time- and cost-effective manner. Efforts to standardize the measurement of hemoglobin A1C—the major indicator of long-term blood glucose control—will help patients to improve their diabetes monitoring and control and, thereby, minimize their risk of developing complications by ensuring that clinical values are comparable to those reported from research studies.

Complications of the eyes, kidneys and urologic tract, nerves, and heart, among other organs, represent a severe health burden for people with diabetes and drive up the costs of health care. The special statutory funding program has a clear focus on understanding the underlying genetics and pathology of complications and on finding new ways to prevent and treat these diabetes-related diseases.

Goal VI: Attract New Talent to Research on Type 1 Diabetes

As is clear from the scope of research being pursued under the other scientific goals of the Special Statutory Funding Program, type 1 diabetes and its complications are extremely complex diseases and span a wide diversity of scientific fields. Moreover, finding effective means to prevent and cure type 1 diabetes requires the dedicated efforts of a continuum of research talent from basic scientists to clinical investigators. A high priority of the program is to attract high-caliber scientists who are applying their specialized expertise and technologies to research on type 1 diabetes.

Bench-to-bedside grants support research collaborations between basic and clinical scientists to rapidly translate discoveries from the laboratory bench to clinical testing in patients. Similarly, innovative partnership grants pair established diabetes investigators with other scientists who can bring needed expertise or research technology to the study of type 1 diabetes. These initiatives support multidisciplinary research that will advance many scientific fields related to type 1 diabetes and its complications. Finally, training and career development programs have been established to encourage the entry of pediatric endocrinologists into a career track in diabetes research.

Attracting new talent and fresh insights as well as utilizing the most up-to-date technology are vital to the advancement of research on the prevention and cure of type 1 diabetes. The special statutory funding program has enabled new approaches to foster the exchange of ideas among scientists and to promote careers in pediatric diabetology. These initiatives will synergize research efforts on this disease and help to bring new research findings to practical use in the type 1 diabetes patient population.

The Special Statutory Funding Program for Type 1 Diabetes Research has stimulated significant scientific advances and the promise of rapid future progress through the support of large-scale research collaborations and diverse investigator-initiated studies. A panel of external scientific and lay experts with respect to type 1 diabetes met in May 2002 at the NIH to assess the program and to identify new opportunities in type 1 diabetes research that have been made possible by the program.

The advisory panel agreed that the special statutory funding program has opened up new research avenues of critical importance to the prevention and cure of type 1 diabetes, including opportunities to:

▷ Understand the role of the Histocompatibility Leukocyte Antigens (HLA), infectious agents, and other potential genetic and environmental factors in the development of type 1 diabetes.

▷ Elucidate the mechanisms of T cell destruction of the beta cells and the role of autoantibodies in this process. Find ways to prevent or reverse the autoimmune process and to preserve residual beta cell function in new onset patients.

▷ Improve and develop new methods for islet transplantation through the use of stem cells, optimized procedures for pancreas harvesting and islet isolation, novel agents for immunosuppression, and advanced transplantation techniques.

▷ Examine the neuronal mechanisms underlying hypoglycemia and hypoglycemia unawareness. Develop new therapies and technologies to counteract hypoglycemia, including improved glucose sensors and insulin delivery devices.

▷ Create new animal models that closely mimic human type 1 diabetes, as well as models for the study of long-term complications. Establish centralized resources for preclinical pharmaceutical testing in animal models and for distributing animals with prolonged hyperglycemia as models of complications.

▷ Develop and apply new reagents and technologies for research on type 1 diabetes diagnosis, prevention, and treatment, including: proteomics approaches, imaging techniques for the pancreas and the brain, synteny and haplotype mapping[6], pathogenic T cell assays, neuronal cell lines, glucose sensors, and microarrays.

▷ Promote interactions, data sharing, and coordination among existing research consortia and establish new, multidisciplinary research groups for the study of hypoglycemia and for collaborative research on multiple, long-term diabetic complications.

▷ Ensure that type 1 diabetes research continues to attract high-caliber research talent to the field. Promote access to state-of-the-art technologies for diabetes research.

The recommendations of the advisory panel will be an important scientific guide to the NIH, CDC, and other HHS components in the development of future initiatives in support of type 1 diabetes research.

6 Synteny mapping is the comparison of DNA sequences among different species to find common genes that may influence disease susceptibility. Haplotype mapping efforts are aimed at finding patterns of genetic variation among humans that are associated with disease.

FUTURE OPPORTUNITIES FOR TYPE 1 DIABETES RESEARCH

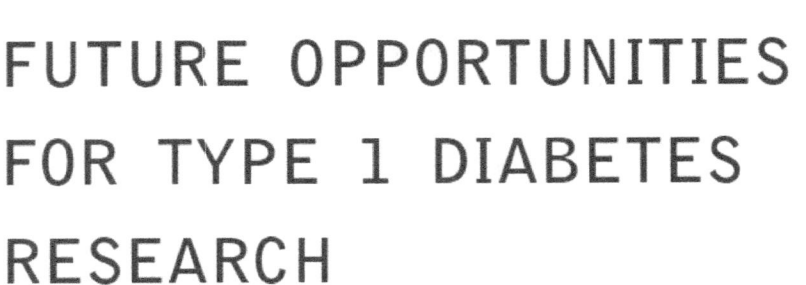

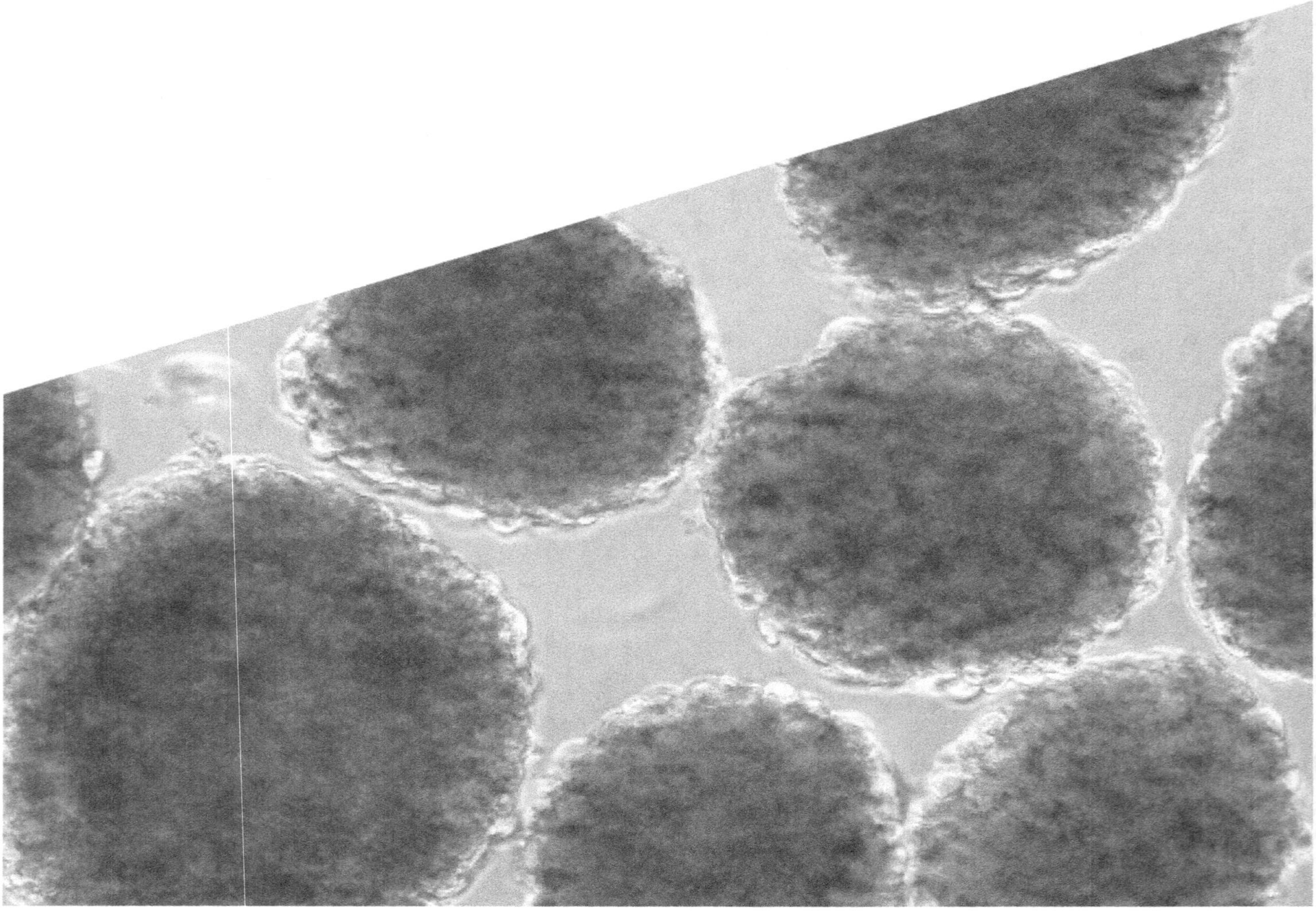

The Special Statutory Funding Program for Type 1 Diabetes Research has supported great strides in the understanding of this disease, but much work remains to be done. Studies to identify how genetic propensities and environmental triggers initiate the disease process in humans are now critical. Continued research on animal and cellular models to understand molecular mechanisms will provide the basis for rational development of preventive agents for type 1 diabetes and its devastating complications. Ongoing investment in clinical trials and research will help scientists translate research advances into real improvements in patients' health. Thus, the research initiatives and resource development projects undertaken with the special funding program to date have sparked exciting new opportunities for future, cutting-edge research on understanding, preventing, and treating type 1 diabetes.

In addition to reviewing the special statutory funding program to date, the advisory panel of leading scientific experts convened at the NIH in May 2002 also assessed accomplishments and considered new research opportunities that have emerged as a result of the program's investment. The panel was encouraged both by the scientific progress supported by the special funds, as well as by the establishment of collaborative research infrastructure, such as consortia and trial networks, that will synergize future research efforts in the field. The advisors' recommendations for future research focused on: new research questions and goals that are critical to continuing advances in type 1 diabetes; the potential to apply new research methodologies to the study of type 1 diabetes; and research resources and infrastructure that would facilitate multidisciplinary approaches to the complex problems of type 1 diabetes and its complications. Following are highlights of specific research opportunities identified by the advisory panel.

Important Questions and Research Goals

- Understand the role of Histocompatibility Leukocyte Antigens (HLA)—which are genetically linked to type 1 diabetes susceptibility—in the development of autoimmunity;

- Define the mechanism of T cell-mediated destruction of the pancreatic beta cells;

- Find methods to reverse autoimmunity by promoting central tolerance and reprogramming of T cells;

- Understand the contributions of autoantibodies to the pathogenesis of type 1 diabetes;

- Identify beta cell antigens that initiate the autoimmune process;

- Examine environmental factors during gestation that potentially modulate future susceptibility to type 1 diabetes;

- Investigate the effect of parental type 1 diabetes on possible immune tolerization of offspring during pregnancy;

- Study infectious agents, including viruses, as possible triggers of the autoimmune reaction leading to type 1 diabetes;

- Use type 1 diabetes as a platform for understanding immunology and autoimmunity.

Applying New Methodologies

- Apply proteomics approaches to the study of insulitis and the identification of circulating beta cell markers;

- Design beta cell imaging technology for use in assessing progression of autoimmune destruction of beta cells;

- Develop assays for identifying pathogenic T cells involved in triggering type 1 diabetes;

- Utilize synteny mapping and haplotype mapping approaches to the identification of genes conferring susceptibility to or protection from development of type 1 diabetes;

- Use PCR-based RNA or DNA analyses to identify infectious agents that may trigger autoimmune diabetes.

Resources and Infrastructure

Devise a system for procurement of pancreata from organ donors, who had been identified as new-onset type 1 patients or autoantibody positive, pre-diabetic individuals, to facilitate research on insulitis—the inflammation of islets by infiltrating T cells;

Promote cross-talk among databases and integration of bioinformatics resources to improve coordination and data-sharing among related consortia and research networks;

Expand the type 1 diabetes animal repository to include non-NOD mouse backgrounds and inbred strains for studies of genetic and environmental susceptibility factors and drug testing;

Establish human sample repositories to facilitate transfer of data and resources among research groups;

Develop new research consortia to expedite the study of genes and environmental factors affecting diabetes susceptibility;

Foster industry collaboration and participation in consortia to bring needed expertise in drug development;

Establish type 1 diabetes as a reportable illness throughout the U.S. to shed light on the magnitude of the type 1 diabetes epidemic.

DNA double helix.

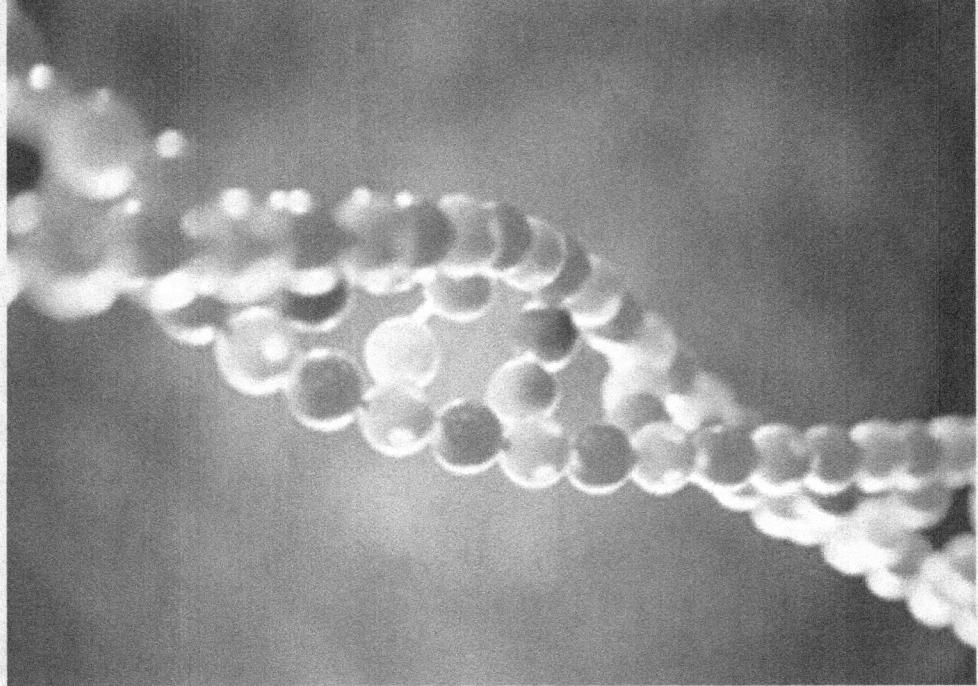

Important Questions and Research Goals

- Develop safe and effective approaches to preventing type 1 diabetes;

- Design methods to preserve or restore residual beta cell function in new-onset patients;

- Improve assays for identifying those at risk of developing type 1 diabetes;

- Generate new technologies for monitoring disease progression.

Applying New Methodologies

- Ensure that pathogenic T cell assays are included in the design of future prevention trials;

- Develop beta cell function assays that can be used as a clinical endpoint sufficient for drug approval.

Resources and Infrastructure

- Establish a central resource to facilitate preclinical studies of new drug efficacy and safety in animals;

- Create "humanized" animal models for the development of more specifically targeted therapies;

- Develop a non-human primate model of autoimmune beta cell destruction that closely mimics the human disease;

- Improve the standardization of C-peptide assays to reduce laboratory variability;

- Enhance human research consortia and interactions;

- Create a centralized Institutional Review Board (IRB) to expedite multi-center clinical trials.

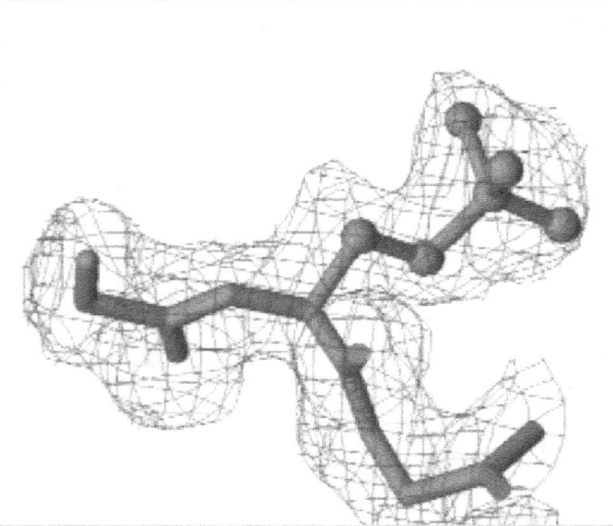

Antibody structure.

Important Questions and Research Goals

- Pursue stem cells or stimulators of stem cells as a source of beta cells that could overcome the short supply of islets available for transplantation by current protocols;

- Delineate the immune components of stem cells as they differentiate to determine whether stem cell-derived replacement beta cells can resist autoimmunity;

- Understand the biology of stressed or injured cells to optimize islet isolation techniques;

- Improve islet transplantation procedures;

- Document risks and benefits of islet transplantation, including issues of cost effectiveness, quality-of-life, and the development of complications.

Applying New Methodologies

- Perform a systematic evaluation of approaches to islet transplantation, including the optimization of:
    pancreas harvesting;
    islet isolation, evaluation, and preservation;
    site and method of islet transplantation;
    immunosuppression, tolerance induction, and other aspects of immunomodulation;

- Apply insights from angiogenesis research to the study of islet graft vascularization;

- Adapt proteomics approaches to measure beta cell specific proteins in plasma for monitoring insulitis and autoimmunity recurrence.

Resources and Infrastructure

- Strengthen mechanisms for data sharing and cross-talk among consortia;

- Expand international collaborations; for example, extend data collection through the islet transplant registry to include international transplantation procedures;

- Improve access to state-of-the-art immunology measurements for transplant trials;

- Explore ongoing opportunities for initiating research support as justified by emerging preliminary data.

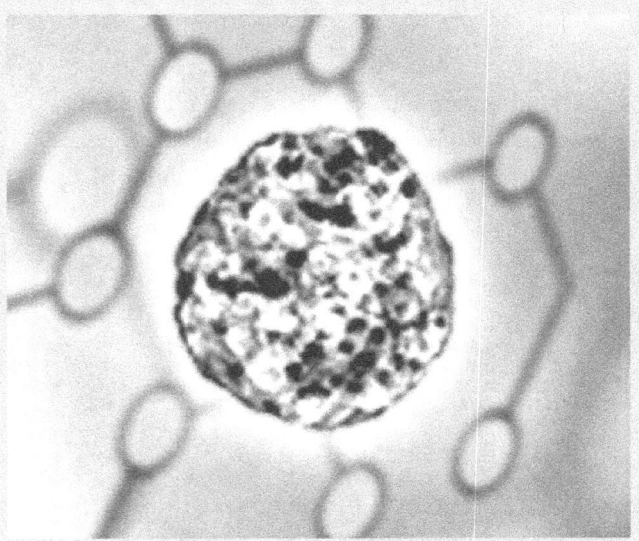

Pancreatic islet.

GOAL IV Prevent or Reduce Hypoglycemia in Type 1 Diabetes

Important Questions and Research Goals

- Understand the mechanisms of hypoglycemia unawareness and nocturnal hypoglycemia;

- Examine the role of glucose transporters and monocarboxylic acid in sensing and responding to hypoglycemia;

- Identify long-term consequences of recurrent hypoglycemia, particularly in young children;

- Develop new therapies, such as insulin analogs, that reduce the occurrence of hypoglycemia;

- Elucidate mechanisms of the reversal of hypoglycemia unawareness and defective counter-regulation to inform the development of pharmaceutical approaches to restore counter-regulation;

- Intensify research on glucose sensors and the development of closed-loop systems for glucose sensing and insulin delivery;

- Evaluate the clinical utility of new glucose sensors and insulin delivery devices, including the effects of these technologies on patients' quality-of-life.

Applying New Methodologies

- Investigate the problem of hypoglycemia unawareness in new islet transplant recipients;

- Recruit neuroscientists and brain-imaging specialists to study similarities in the glucose-sensing mechanisms of the pancreatic beta cells and the brain;

- Develop neuronal cell lines for the study of glucose sensing;

- Use new sensors that measure neurotransmitter substrates in the brain for investigation of brain glucose sensing;

- Use MRI spectroscopy, brain volume measurement, and other advanced imaging technologies to identify brain changes after recurrent and/or severe hypoglycemia;

- Apply new glucose sensor technology to the development of methods for metabolic screening in research animals.

Resources and Infrastructure

- Establish multidisciplinary research consortia to foster new approaches to the problem of hypoglycemia.

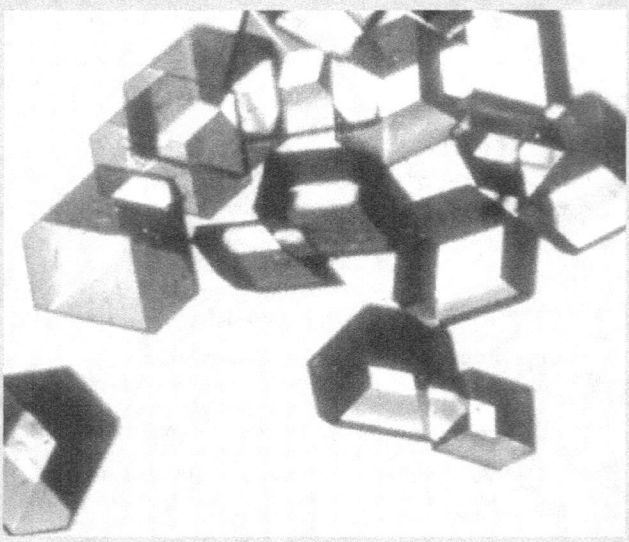

Insulin crystals.

GOAL V Prevent or Reduce Complications of Type 1 Diabetes

Important Questions and Research Goals

Uncover the role of inflammation in vascular complications of diabetes, particularly with respect to the functional interactions between monocytes and endothelial cells;

Expand clinical studies of the role of aspirin, statin therapy, blood pressure control, and other factors, which are effective in preventing cardiovascular disease in type 2 diabetes, to type 1 diabetes;

Develop improved animal models of diabetes complications.

Applying New Methodologies

Use monocytes for assessing the effects of interventions that affect inflammatory pathways relevant to vascular complications;

Develop microarrays for research on gene expression patterns in tissues and organs affected by diabetic complications;

Use congenic technology to develop rat and mouse models that combine diabetic susceptibility with the propensity to develop long-term complications.

Resources and Infrastructure

Form consortia of investigators studying individual complications to promote tissue sharing and examination of multiple complications—particularly in studies of new therapeutic agents in humans and animals—to enhance the cost effectiveness of research;

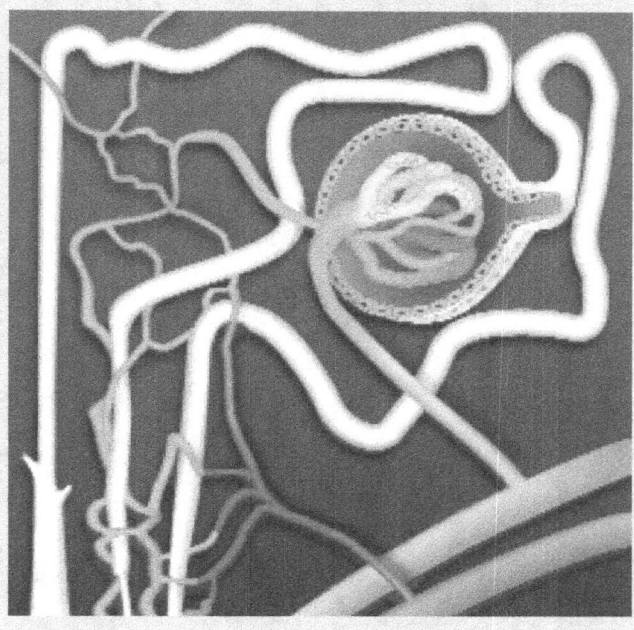

Kidney nephron diagram.

(Credit: Maryetta Lancaster, for NIH Medical Arts and Photography Branch).

Establish consortia of endothelial cell biologists, immunologists, and investigators studying inflammation to study cardiovascular disease in type 1 diabetes;

Encourage partnerships between industry and academia to spur drug development and testing;

Develop mechanisms to bring discoveries with therapeutic applications that originate in academic laboratories through preclinical development;

Create a resource for distributing animals with prolonged, sustained hyperglycemia for use in testing new therapeutics;

Publish a central knowledge base of complications-related initiatives supported across the NIH.

Important Questions and Research Goals

▶ Attract new basic and clinical researchers to research on type 1 diabetes;

▶ Ensure that new technologies and insights from a variety of fields are rapidly applied to research on type 1 diabetes.

Resources and Infrastructure

▶ Extend opportunities for research training and pilot and feasibility studies beyond the life span of a single solicitation;

▶ Issue flexible solicitations that allow investigators to identify promising projects from a breadth of research areas.

Public Health Service grant application.

(Photo Credit: Richard Nowitz for NIDDK)

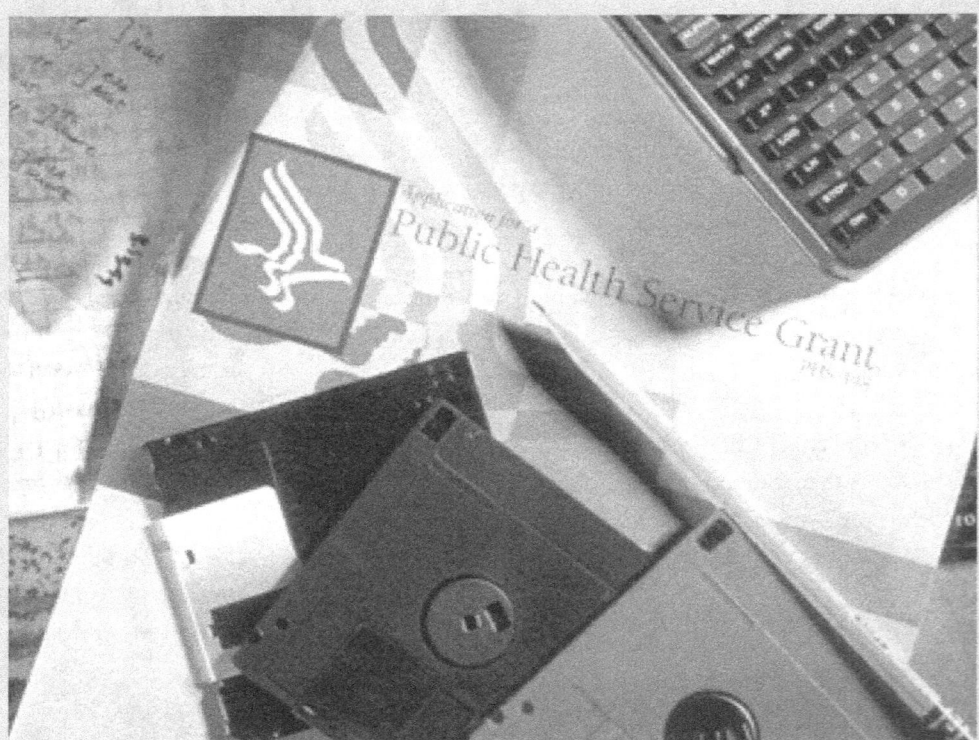

PRODUCTION CREDITS

Evaluation and Production Coordinator
Michelle A. Cissell, PhD, NIDDK Office of Scientific
Program and Policy Analysis

Financial Data
Charles Zellers, NIDDK Office of Financial
Management and Analysis

Design
Joe Vuthipong, Computercraft

Logistical Support
Khari Shamba and Joan Starr, NIDDK Office of Scientific
Program and Policy Analysis